Dainara Danila Nápoles Pastoriza
Alejandro Hernández Niubo
Gloria Marina Fonseca Lloga

Stom-VIH-Soft a tool for learning about HIV/AIDS

Dainara Danila Nápoles Pastoriza
Alejandro Hernández Niubo
Gloria Marina Fonseca Lloga

Stom-VIH-Soft a tool for learning about HIV/AIDS

and its relationship to medical care in Oral Surgery

ScienciaScripts

Imprint

Cover image: www.ingimage.com

This book is a translation from the original published under ISBN 978-613-9-40543-5.

Publisher:
Sciencia Scripts
is a trademark of
Dodo Books Indian Ocean Ltd. and OmniScriptum S.R.L publishing group

120 High Road, East Finchley, London, N2 9ED, United Kingdom
Str. Armeneasca 28/1, office 1, Chisinau MD-2012, Republic of Moldova, Europe
Managing Directors: Ieva Konstantinova, Victoria Ursu
info@omniscriptum.com

Printed at: see last page
ISBN: 978-620-8-52954-3

University of Medical Sciences Faculty of Stomatology

Stom-VIH-Soft a tool for learning about HIV/AIDS and its relationship to medical care in Oral Surgery. and its relationship with medical care in Oral Surgery.

Dainara Danila Nápoles Pastoriza

D. in Stomatology. 3rd year resident of Maxillofacial Surgery.

Alejandro Hernández Niubo

Dr. in Stomatology. Specialist in 1st Degree of General Comprehensive Stomatology.

Gloria Marina Fonseca Lloga

Dr. in Stomatology. Specialist in 1st Degree of General Comprehensive Stomatology. 2nd Year Maxillofacial Surgery Resident

SUMMARY

Introduction: At present HIV/AIDS is a serious problem affecting Cuba and especially the province of Santiago de Cuba, maxillofacial surgeons play a key role in terms of detection, prevention, treatment for it the academic training of the stomatologist and maxillofacial surgeon needs to integrate knowledge acquired in different subjects, which is why the realization and application of new techniques to support teaching such as teaching materials is imposed.

Objective: To develop a didactic material to support the teaching-educational process for the Stomatology course that integrates the fundamental knowledge about HIV/AIDS and its relation to medical care in oral surgery.

Methodological Design: A technological innovation type research was conducted in the Faculty of Stomatology of Santiago de Cuba in the period from January to April 2018, aimed at students of terminal years For the preparation of the educational hyperenvironment the programs CrheaSoft 3.3.3, Paint, Photoshop, Microsoft Office PowerPoint and WondersharePhotoStoryPlatinum were used.

Results: Most of the students preferred the educational hyperenvironment as a didactic teaching medium. This was made with the title of Estom-VIH- Soft and its application increased to 93.3% of the students with an adequate level of knowledge and was valued by 100% of the specialists as a means of practical usefulness.

Conclusions: The Estom-VIH-Soft educational hyperenvironment was designed that integrates the fundamental contents related to HIV-AIDS and its relation to practice in oral surgery.

Key words: educational hyperenvironment, HIV-AIDS, oral surgery.

INDEX

INTRODUCTION

The emergence of HIV infection and AIDS has made a perennial impact on humanity. AIDS is not just a disease, but the final stage of HIV infection, characterized by a set of potentially fatal diseases. More than 20 years have passed since the causative agent was identified and even though progress has been made in differentiating its characteristics and mechanism of infection, no effective treatment has been discovered to cure the disease [1].

In 2016 ,36.7 million people were living with HIV worldwide, 1.8 million people contracted HIV infection ,1 million people died from AIDS-related illnesses,76.1 million people contracted HIV infection since the beginning of the epidemic and 35.0 million people died from AIDS-related illnesses since the beginning of the epidemic [2].

Currently in Cuba there is a large increase in the total number of people living with HIV/AIDS especially in the Province of Santiago de Cuba where as of April 11, 2018 there were a total of 2 262 cases of HIV being the male sex the most affected 80% and men who have sex with men, being also the municipality of Santiago de Cuba the one with the highest prevalence of the disease where the health sector occupies the second position according to the accumulated incidence by sectors [2].

It is essential to always keep in mind the important role played by stomatologists and maxillofacial surgeons as part of the health personnel in charge of the specialized care needed by these patients, also taking into account that oral infectious diseases affect HIV-infected people during all stages the disease, so they may be the first to recognize the signs and symptoms that occur in HIV-AIDS infection, which are common and include new presentations of opportunistic diseases recognized as such (3- 5).

The training of stomatology professionals in Cuba should fundamentally respond to the health needs of both the country and the province, and the efficient and timely care of patients with HIV is a current priority for the country and the province of Santiago de Cuba. .

The subject of HIV-AIDS and its relation to medical care in oral surgery includes elements of promotion, prevention, diagnosis, b i o s e g u r i t y , surgical treatment and medical ethics, which are very necessary for the professional work of the oral surgeon who will require the necessary tools to identify, diagnose, treat and refer to other specialties required [3,6].

The academic training of the stomatologist in oral surgery requires the integration of knowledge acquired in different subjects, that is to say, interdisciplinarity.

This is why it is necessary to develop and apply new techniques to consolidate and integrate the essential knowledge needed by professionals in medical science careers, particularly in Stomatology.

The solution to this problem could be found in the use of dynamic and simple means to support teaching. The different teaching techniques and means to be used for the execution of educational actions constitute a set of procedures aimed modifying knowledge, attitudes and practices, as well as raising awareness of health problems, both individually and collectively [7-9].

With the teaching aids, the potentialities that our sense organs have for learning are used to a greater extent; on average, a normal person learns: through taste 1%, touch 1.5%, through smell 3.5%, through hearing 11.0% and through sight 83.0% (10,11).

In their application, imagination and creativity are needed to be able to modify and adapt knowledge according to the participants and the specific situation to be faced (12). according to the participants and the specific situation be faced [12].

After carrying out an extensive search through INFOMED to find out the existence of any digital product that integrated all the elements related to HIV/AIDS and its relation to medical care in oral surgery, it was found that were few other products on this subject.

Scientific Problem:

Taking into account that on several occasions the students of the Stomatology career have raised the need to increase the support materials that integrate the contents, mainly in the final years of the career where the ability to integrate the contents taught in previous years and in different subjects becomes more complex, and due to the relevance that the topic of HIV-AIDS has at present for the province of Santiago de Cuba, the following question was posed:

How to contribute to the integration of fundamental knowledge about HIV/AIDS and its relationship with medical care in oral surgery during the educational teaching process of the Stomatology career in order to increase knowledge about this topic?

Justification of the study:

The medical sciences are undergoing a pedagogical revolution as a result of the transformations that have occurred in the process of universalization of teaching. The use of an Educational Software of hyper educational environment type favors the presence in the classrooms of a more creative student, who participates more actively facilitating the teaching-learning and the integration of knowledge. Given the need that exists in stomatology students who face a universalization where the use of didactic materials is required, which compile explicit information, previously reviewed and sometimes difficult to access to the student, the need arises to establish an automated digital bridge that would be the software, that enhances a good doctor-patient relationship for the provision of quality stomatological and maxillofacial medical care in terms of diagnosis, prognosis and treatment plan, mainly to patients who require comprehensive and efficient care, as is the case of people living with HIV-AIDS.

Hypothesis: If a didactic means of support to the teaching-educational process that integrates the fundamental knowledge about HIV/AIDS and its relation medical care in oral surgery is developed, students' knowledge about this topic will be increased.

GENERAL OBJECTIVE:

To prepare a didactic material to support the teaching-educational process for the Stomatology course that integrates the fundamental knowledge about HIV/AIDS and its relation to medical care in oral surgery.

SPECIFIC OBJECTIVES:

1- To assess the level of knowledge of the students selected for the study this topic.

2- Identify the teaching medium preferred by students for learning the subject matter in .

3- Design the teaching medium preferred by students for the study of the subject.

4- To verify the scientific value of the designed medium through the evaluation of the students' knowledge after interacting with the product and its assessment by users and specialists.

METHODOLOGICAL DESIGN

In order to carry out this research, it was necessary, in an initial stage, to conduct a detailed investigation of the subjects taught in the courses of Microbiology, Oral Medicine I, Periodontics, Oral Surgery, Oral Medicine II, in order to students of Stomatology career, as well as to study the objectives set out in the plan D for the subjects, under the advice and supervision of the tutor.

DESIGN OF THE FINISHED PRODUCT:

Place and period in which the product was manufactured:

Faculty of Stomatology of Santiago de Cuba, during the period from January to April 2018.

Type of research:

Technological innovation. The selected product was an educational hyperenvironment

Personnel involved and tasks assigned: Three researchers participated:

Dr. Dainara Danila Nápoles Pastoriza

Dr.Alejandro Hernández Niubo

Dr. Gloria Marina Fonseca Lloga

They carried out the design of the teaching media, as well as the search and compilation of the information, and prepared the final report of the product.

Elements used in the manufacture of the product:

An ASUS computer was used in the design. Intel(R)Caleron(R) CPU N3050@ 1.60GHz.

Operating System: Windows 10 Home Single Language

CrheaSoft 3.3.3 was used. **CrheaSoft 3.3.3**: This is used to create Flash, HTML, EXE and CD-ROM presentations. Its interface is as easy to use as drag and drop, with no programming skills . It uses an icon-based development system. Each icon is equivalent to an element that can be integrated into the project, whether it is a text, an image or a video. CrheaSoft 3.3.3 is characterized by allowing the configuration of events for the different objects that make up a project. It is a necessary tool to create presentations with special effects, as well as to present work with variables and the use of Scripts, and it allows to add files in different formats such as Word, PDF, Power Point and compacted files.

Adobe Photoshop 10 CS3 Portable: Professional program used for image editing, as well as the creation of backgrounds and buttons.

Microsoft Office 2016: Package used for processing the text contained in the hyperenvironment and elaboration of tables and graphs of the research report **Main procedures by means which the product was designed**:

The educational hyperenvironment was developed in three stages:

1- Search and compilation of information: The information contained in this product was obtained through several updated books and journals on the subject; all the bibliography consulted is set out in this report.

2- Selection of the tools for its creation: after evaluating several tools for the creation of the educational hyperenvironment, it was decided to use CrheaSoft 3.3.3. Adobe Photoshop 10 CS3 Portable and Microsoft Office 2016, Pro Show Gold 3.2 and Ulead Video Studio 10.

3- Product design: It was designed to facilitate motivation, learning new knowledge and deepening previous knowledge, providing new stimuli and activating the students' response system. In addition, it was aimed at providing updated information and resources to improve the quality of teaching, and visual effects were generated and related to the digital environment. In this design stage, the textual content, animations and images, the hyperenvironment environment and the logical structure of its operation were elaborated, based programming resources. It was decided that the graphics, animations and images would be created following the format and style of color ranges and shades conceived according to the design.

Minimum requirements for running the product on a computer:

- Intel Celeron(R) 1.2 GHz microprocessor
- Operating system Windows 2000 and higher
- 256MB of RAM
- CD-ROM-DVD

Requirements for its use:

- Maintenance Requirements: The system does not require maintenance.
- Reliability Requirements: It is reliable, accurate, and practically free of faults.
- Performance Requirements: Good performance, good speed, and good response time.
- Hardware Platform Requirements: PC: Pentium III at 1.0 GHz and 256 MB of RAM.
- Software Platform Requirements: Operating System Windows 2000 and higher.
- Ease of Learning: Learning to navigate the hyperenvironment is easy and fast.

DESIGN OF THE VERIFICATION STUDY:

A technological innovation type study was carried out, consisting of the creation of an educational hyperenvironment, which contains all the necessary information that integrates the fundamental knowledge on HIV/AIDS medical care in oral surgery for students in the final years of the Stomatology career (mainly 5th year).

The study was conducted at the Faculty of Stomatology of Santiago de Cuba in the period from January to April 2018.

For this stage, a questionnaire was administered to the fifth-year stomatology students (Annex 2), thus forming a quasi-experimental before-after study without a control group.

Definition of the Study Universe

It was constituted by the 5th year students of the Stomatology career in Santiago de Cuba in the period from January to April 2018 for a total of 130, selecting a sample of 30 students through simple random sampling.

Inclusion criteria: 5th year students of the Stomatology Career of Santiago de Cuba who gave their informed consent to participate in the research.

Exclusion criteria: 5th year students of the Stomatology Career of Santiago de Cuba who request leave of absence due to illness or any other cause.

The research was carried out in 4 stages:

First Stage:

The participants in the study were given an initial diagnostic test (Annex 1) related to the topic in question, without the use of the teaching medium, in order to check levels of knowledge, according to the aforementioned selection criteria.

Operationalization of the Variable:

Variable	Ranking	Scale
Knowledge level	Qualitative ordinal Polytomous	Adequate Moderately adequate Inadequate

Adequate: More than 80% of the questions answered correctly.

Moderately adequate: Between 60 and 80% of the questions answered correctly.

Inadequate: Less than 60% of the questions answered correctly.

-A questionnaire was prepared (Annex 2), in which the preference of how to receive HIV/AIDS information and its relation to medical care in oral surgery was collected the students who participated in the research, offering the student a series of suitable educational means to be selected. It should be noted that during the application of the survey, it was explained to the students what each medium consisted of in case there were any doubts related to them.

Operationalization of the Variable:

Variable	**Ranking**	**Scale**
Means of preference for gain knowledge	Qualitative Nominal Qualitative Polytomous	Educational hyperenvironment Audiovisual program Website PowerPoint with hyperlinks

These data allowed us to know the preferences the students of the Stomatology career in terms of how to receive the information, which were taken into account for the design of the didactic media.

Second Stage:

Once the hyperenvironment was prepared, it was submitted to the criteria of specialists. These were specialists with experience in the subject of HIV/AIDS and its relationship with medical care in oral surgery and in Computer Sciences, teachers of the career of Stomatology. Their selection was determined by means of a non-probabilistic purposive sampling (sampling by criteria), considering the following criteria:

Inclusion criteria:

- Have knowledge and experience in the subject.
- To be an IT specialist.
- Have teaching status.

- Willingness to participate in the testing of the software product.

Taking into consideration the above criteria, a sample of 4 specialists was selected:

- 2 specialists in II Degree of General Comprehensive Stomatology and Maxillofacial Surgery, with experience in the care of patients with HIV.
- 2 specialists in Computer Science

This group of specialists filled out a questionnaire (Annex 3).

Operationalization of Variable:

Variable	Ranking	Scale
Presentation Quality	Qualitative Ordinal polytomous	High Medium Low
Quality of production	Qualitative Ordinal polytomous	High Medium Low
Scientific quality	Qualitative Ordinal polytomous	High Medium Low
Practical Utility	Qualitative ordinal ordinal polytomous	Total Partial None

Third Stage:

The level of knowledge of the students was evaluated after they interacted with the designed teaching medium, taking into account the same variable and scale used in the first stage to measure knowledge.

Fourth Stage:

Evaluation of the educational hyperenvironment by 5th year students of the Stomatology Career in Santiago de Cuba (Annex 4).

Operationalization of the variables:

Variable	Ranking	Scale
Ease of use and interaction	Qualitative ordinal Polytomous	Total Partial None

Quality of images, videos and simulations sound	Qualitative Ordinal Polytomous	High Medium Low
Level of understanding of the content	Qualitative Ordinal Polytomous	Adequate Adequate Moderately adequate Inadequate
Design and Colors	Qualitative Ordinal Polytomous	Adequate Adequate Moderately adequate Inadequate
Help to integrate knowledge	Qualitative ordinal Polytomous	Total Partial None
Motivation	Qualitative Nominal Dichotomous	Yes No
Acceptability of employment as a teaching	Qualitative Nominal Dichotomous	Accepted Not accepted

Procedures and techniques to collect information:

The information was obtained from the completion of the surveys where it appears what was expressed by the students and specialists. Each student was allowed 45 minutes for the resolution of the questions in the case of diagnostics. These questions were designed according to the knowledge that the students should have on the subject, according to the program.

Processing and analysis:

The data was processed on an ASUS computer. Intel(R)Caleron(R) CPU N3050@ 1.60GHz, with the Windows 10 Home Single Language operating system. With the data obtained after the application of the survey to the students, several data bases were made in the SPSS program version 21.0, which allowed the application of the pertinent statistical calculations, the percentage analysis was carried out and tables of absolute frequencies and percentages are presented, which offer a better understanding.

Ethical aspects

In order to carry out the study, the approval of the directors of the institution where the teaching method was used was requested (Appendix 5), the confidentiality of criteria and the moral integrity of the participants was guaranteed, and approval to participate was requested by means of an informed consent form (Appendix 6).

DEVELOPMENT

The product developed was an educational hyperenvironment entitled: **Estom-VIH-Soft. Characteristics of the educational hyperenvironment.**

Integrates essential theoretical and practical knowledge on the subject. Maintains student motivation.

Presents important and current information on the subject. user interaction with the application

Structure and operation of Estom-VIH-Soft

The product is structured by modules and each of these can be accessed at any time during navigation, maintaining the same access options at all times through a top menu, some modules will have their own particular navigation according to their different functionalities.

All products will be started in the enlarged screen, to restore to normal screen it is done through the F11 button on the keyboard.

In the upper right part of the product you will find the close button X . Clicking on it will close the product together with the server.

Relevant product data will be displayed on the home page.

Module Syllabus (Annex 7)

The Topics module displays a drop-down window with the Table of Contents that includes 7 sections: Epidemiology of HIV/AIDS, History of the disease, HIV/AIDS diagnosis and prevention, Oral manifestations of HIV/AIDS, Biosafety and HIV/AIDS, Oral surgical treatment in patients with HIV/AIDS, Methodological instrument for comprehensive dental care for people living with HIV/AIDS, and Ethical aspects of care for patients with HIV/AIDS.

When selecting the tab **Subject**, the screen shows a **drop-down window** with the **Table of Contents** with all the topics and subtopics for reading that exist, each topic can have subtopics, and these will be shown by clicking on the topic and all the subtopics it has will be displayed just below. The topics or subtopics that have content to read will be displayed with an icon at on the side. To visualize this content, press the button , automatically the drop-down window will be hidden and the content will be shown.

By clicking on the icon ( ) at any time, the **drop-down window** will be picked up and displayed as appropriate.

At the bottom right of the screen where the content is displayed, there is a paging bar with the number of pages that exist and the number of the current page, as well as different options to navigate through the pages.

Hyperlinks to different Topics or Subtopics will appear in the content and will be displayed in blue. Clicking on this will take you to the destination of the hyperlink.

Module Exercise (Annex 8)

The Exercises module leads to the corresponding page, which has a series of questions that will make the user investigate and integrate knowledge, from the deepening of the contents exposed, which makes this page one of the most relevant of the Hyperenvironment, with modalities such as true or false.
complete and in the form of clinical cases

In this module you will be able to train through a system of already elaborated exercises, for this you must make a selection of the exercises you wish to perform. A list with all the existing topics will be displayed on the screen, where you can select the ones you want by clicking on the corresponding button. If you wish to do all the topics, the option **All** appears at the bottom of the box.

On the right side there are two options **Intervals** and **Assigned**. With these options the user can choose the exercises and the way he/she wants to perform them.

By **Intervals**

Once you have selected the topic(s) in which the training will be performed, the number of exercises in each topic is displayed. A **Start** and **End** interval is shown. The latter will show the maximum number of exercises. This interval can be modified as the user wishes, taking into account that it does not exceed the maximum number of exercises.

Next, two options **Sequential** and **Random** appear.

If the **Sequential** option is selected, the exercises will appear consecutively. To start performing the exercises, click on the **Start** button at the bottom right. In the case of the **Random** option, initially the total amount of the topic is shown, this amount depends on the number of exercises that the user wants to do, regardless of the number and type of question. To start the go to the **Start** button the bottom right.

Once the exercise system has been started, a bar is displayed at the bottom of the screen. bar with different options. On the left side navigation options (first exercise, previous exercise, next exercise, last exercise and exit the trainer) as well as the number of exercises to be performed and the position of the current exercise.

Selecting the **Exit Trainer** button 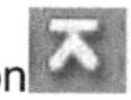 will display a confirmation window asking if you want to Exit the training. If you want to exit go to the
OK button. Otherwise go to the **Cancel** button.

At the bottom right are the **Finish**, **Review** buttons and an icon
Help.

If the **Finish** button is clicked, the exercise is terminated and a screen with the **Training Results** and statistics is displayed.

If you wish to save the results obtained in the training, click on the **Save Result** button at the bottom of the screen. This operation must be done before **exiting the training**, because once you are out of the training you will not be able to obtain the results.

In the case of selecting the **Review** button, a window appears with the remaining attempts to be made. When all the attempts are exhausted, two new buttons appear in the lower right part of the window: **Your Answer** and **Correct Answer**. Selecting the **Your Answer** button displays the last answer given by the user. Selecting the **Correct Answer** button will display the correct answer.

If the **Help** button is selected, a window with a Guidance for the Question appears. To exit click on the **OK** button.

The training is not finished until you click on the **Exit** button **of the**

Trainer located in the bottom bar of the screen. A message will appear warning the user if he/she really wants to exit, if yes, click on the **Ok** button, if no, click on the **Ok** button, if no, click on the **Ok** button, if no, click on the **Ok** button.

On the contrary, click on the **Cancel** button in the **Media Library Module** (Annex 9).

In this module you will have access to different media. To access these, just move the mouse pointer over the **Media Library** tab and a menu with the existing galleries (images, videos, sounds and animation) will be displayed. When selecting one of the galleries, the structure by categories will be loaded on the left side of the screen. This hyperenvironment has updated videos and images related to the subject matter, some videos in English to complement the current curricular strategy of the English language in medical science careers.

On the right side of the screen all loaded socks are displayed according to the selected category, at the beginning first category will be displayed by default. When passing

If you hover the mouse pointer over the mean, a description of the mean will be displayed, and by clicking on the mean, the will be played on the screen.

Complement Module

This module will show all bibliographies and bibliographic complements distributed by categories. To access these complements, after selecting the **Complement** tab**,** a list of all the categories will be displayed on the left side and by selecting one of them, the files it contains will be displayed on the right side, with representative icons of each material with the possibility of downloading them at any time.

Games Module

In the **Hangman** game (Annex 10)

Select the level of complexity you wish to play.

- Level 1: offers the orientation of the exercise, the question referring to the word and the first letter of the word to be guessed.
- Level 2: provides the orientation of the exercise and the question concerning the word.
- Level 3: does not offer any information and is played against time.

In this module, as in the exercises, the student has the opportunity to learn by playing, to apply the knowledge they have on the subject, it is especially recommended to motivate those less interested in the subject, because through a different and unconventional way within the teaching process, they are brought closer to the knowledge.

Help module Methodological help:

This help will show guidance made by the product developer for the user using the software.

VERIFICATION STUDY RESULTS

Table 1. Level of knowledge before and after the use of the Estom-VIH-Soft product. Faculty of Stomatology of Santiago de Cuba. 2018.

Moment	Knowledge level					
	Suitable		Moderately appropriate		Inadequate	
	No	%	No	%	No	%
Formerly	2	6,6	4	13,3	24	80
Then	28	93,3	1	3,3	1	3,3

*Calculated based on the total number of students surveyed.

Before the students interacted with the product, 80% of them had an inadequate level of knowledge and after the application of the product, 93.3% of them had an adequate level of knowledge.

Table 2. Students' preferred means of receiving information on the subject.

Means of obtaining knowledge	**No**	**%***
Educational hyperenvironment	29	96,6
Websites	1	3,3
Power point with hyperlink	0	0
Audiovisual program	0	0

96.6% of the students selected the educational hyperenvironment as their preferred means of obtaining information on the subject.

Table 3. Assessment of hyperenvironment according to specialists' criteria.

Aspects to evaluate	**Evaluation**	**No**	**%***
Presentation Quality	High	3	75
	Media	1	25
	Download	0	0

Quality of production	High	4	100
	Media	0	0
	Download	0	0
Quality of content	High	4	100
	Media	0	0
	Download	0	0
Practical utility	Total	4	100
	Partial	0	0
	None	0	0

**Calculated based on the total number of specialists.

100% of the specialists concluded that the quality of the content of the hyperenvironment was high and that it was of great practical use.

Table 4. Evaluation of the hyperenvironment according to students' criteria

Aspects to evaluate	**Evaluation**	**No**	**%**
Ease of use and interaction	Total	29	96,6
	Partial	1	3,3
	None	0	0
Quality of images, videos and sound simulations	Ata	30	100
	Media	0	0
	Download	0	0
Understanding the content	Adequate	30	100
	Moderately adequate	0	0
	Inadequate	0	0
Design and Colors	Suitable	28	93,3
	Moderately adequate	2	6,6
	Inadequate	0	0
Help to integrate the content	Total	30	100
	Partial	0	0
	None	0	0

*

100% of the students considered that the quality of the images and videos was high, that the comprehension of the content was adequate and that the hyperenvironment helps to integrate the content fully.

Table 5. Students' level of satisfaction with the hyperenvironment.

Acceptability of its use as a medium of education	**No**	**%***
Accepted	30	100
Not accepted	0	0

*

100% of the students accepted the use of the hyperenvironment as a teaching aid to support teaching.

Table 6. Students' motivation with the hyperenvironment.

Motivation	**No**	**%***
Yes	30	100
No	0	0

*

100% of the students' students felt motivated with the hyperenvironment.

DISCUSSION

The hyperenvironment Stom-HIV-Soft. as didactic material to support teaching allows consolidating, integrating and applying in a practical way the knowledge about HIV/AIDS and its relation with medical attention in oral surgery, of vital importance for the integral formation of students as future Stomatology professionals.

Educational hyper-environments are a great attraction for educational establishments, which see their presentations as a useful teaching tool. They must be above all, endowed with dynamism so that the youngest students put all their attention on them and the learning process is a success. [13]

After multimedia was made, it was submitted to the evaluation of specialists, where the practical usefulness of the product in this research turned out to be the most valued variable, being equal the opinion of all specialists regarding the benefit that the implementation of the material represents in the career, since they state that it constitutes a didactic alternative of support for the teaching-educational process.

After the students interacted with the product, a significant increase in knowledge related to the subject matter was observed with respect to the results obtained in the initial diagnosis, results that contribute to support the quality and effectiveness of the teaching tool in question.

A hyperenvironment is based on the dialogue between users and content, where design and realization (audiovisual media) are the main factors to capture their attention, since success depends on the person, receiver or user being able to fully relate to the presentation [13], an aspect that was achieved with this product since the vast majority students evaluated that these elements had a high quality, achieving the transmission of the message, which facilitates and stimulates the review of its content, allowing the practical application of the knowledge acquired and the development of skills.

Another aspect to bear in mind is that the topic addressed not only has an important impact on the current panorama of the country and the province of Santiago de Cuba, but also constitutes a topic whose bibliographic content is very wide, which is dispersed in different subjects of the Stomatology career and for this reason it is often more difficult for students to integrate all the contents, which is why this hyperenvironment not only integrates the contents established in the study plan regarding the topic of HIV/AIDS and its relation to medical care in oral surgery, It also helps to avoid the dissemination of information obtained through the network or by using foreign software, which should be purchased and would mean an unnecessary economic expense. All these aspects were well achieved since all the students who participated said that the hyperenvironment provided them with total help to integrate the contents, Moreover, the importance of the product is based on this aspect, since in the country there have been many multimedia related to HIV/AIDS prevention, such as the one carried out by the authors Estévez Solano and Bravo de las Casas [14], as well as others more related to the career of medicine, But very few products related to stomatology and oral surgery, and in the search made on the Internet, none was found in this province that integrated all the aspects of the study plan related to this topic but that also went beyond the oral manifestations of this pathology and that managed to reflect other important aspects of oral surgical treatment as well the educational intervention program aimed at people living with HIV, which is the basis of much of the stomatological care of these patients in Cuba.

Authors such as Monteagudo [15] recommend the use of educational software in topics related to HIV/AIDS; in addition, its use in university teaching and especially in health students favors student motivation and, therefore, increases the possibilities of greater learning, an aspect that was achieved with the creation of this product since all students reported feeling motivated with the Estom-VIH-Soft educational hyperenvironment.

CONCLUSIONS

The Estom-VIH-Soft educational hyperenvironment was designed to integrate the fundamental contents related to HIV-AIDS and its relationship with medical care in oral surgery, achieving an increase in knowledge related to the subject after the interaction of students with the software compared to the results obtained in initial diagnosis applied to them.

RECOMMENDATIONS

It is recommended to generalize the product with all students, as well as to extend its its use not only to undergraduate but also to postgraduate.

REFERENCES BIBLIOGRAPHIC REFERENCES

1- Murillo Ladinez N Y. Acute Ulcerative Necrotizing Lesions and their relationship HIV/AIDS [doctoral thesis]. Guayaquil: University of Guayaquil. Pilot Faculty of Dentistry ;2014

2- HIV and AIDS. Statistical data. Infomed. 2017. [cited 17 March 2018]. Available from: http://temas.sld.cu/vihsida/informacion-basica/sobre-vih-y- aids/statistical-data/summary-2017/.

3- Alemán Miranda O, Jardón Caballero J, Domínguez Y. Infectology and parasites in Stomatology [monograph on the Internet]. Madrid: Editorial Académica Española ;2017. [cited 10 March 2018]. Available from: https://www.amazon.es/Infectología-y-parásitos-en

Estomatología/dp/6202235594

4- Gallardo-Rosales R, Castillo-Torres K, Alegría-Conejeros P, Blackburn- Tapia E. Oral manifestations in HIV/AIDS patients at the Base Hospital of Valdivia in Chile. Rev CES Odont [journal on the Internet] 2016. [cited 17 March 2018]; 29(2): 12-19. Available inwww.scielo.org.co/pdf/ceso/v29n2/v29n2a03.pdf

5- Alemán Miranda O, Jardón Caballero J, Domínguez Y. Oral conditions related to HIV/AIDS. [monograph on the Internet]. Madrid: Editorial Academica Española ;2017. [cited 17 March 2018]. Available from: https://www.amazon.es/Afecciones-bucodentales-relacionadas-VIH-SIDA/.../3330091.

6- Alemán Miranda O, Domínguez Y, Aput A. Biosafety in HIV/AIDS. [monograph on the Internet]. Madrid: Editorial Academica Española ;2017. [cited 10 March 2018]. Available from:

https://www.amazon.es/Bioseguridad-SIDA-Otto-Alemán- Miranda/dp/6202249889

7- Sierras Gómez, M. [cited 17 March 2018]. Design of didactic media and resources [monograph on the Internet] Madrid: Innovación y cualificación; 2012 [cited. 15 March 2018].Available from: https://books.google.com.cu/books?id=1Hlbqe31EncC&pg=PA9&lpg=PA9&dq= Innovaci%C3%B3n+y+cualificaci%C3%B3n.+Design%C3%B1o+of+means+and+re+ did%C3%A1ctical+courses&source=bl&ots=kgoq5GIkNI&sig=- flpUncUzA1v9r0ESF_Znopy0q4&hl=en- 419&sa=X&ved=2ahUKEwiamsbq34HeAhVwqlkKHQ3PDGYQ6AEwCnoECAQ QAQ#v=onepage&q=Innovation%C3%B3n%20and%20qualification%C3%B3n.%20 Di se%C3%B1o%20de%20medios%20y%20recursos%20did%C3%A1cticos&f=fa lse

8- Ruiz Piedra AM, Gómez Martínez F. Educational software and ethical principles. Educ Méd Super [Journal on the Internet] 2013 [cited March 6, 2018]; 27(2): 160-5. Available from: http://www.ems.sld.cu/index.php/ems/article/view/161/84

9- Díaz del Mazo L, Ferrer González S, García Díaz R, Duarte Escalante A. Changes in oral health knowledge and attitudes in adolescents from Reparto Sueño. MEDISAN [Journal on the Internet] 2001 [cited 3 February 2018]; 5(2): 4-7 .Available. at: http://www.bus.sld.cu/revistas/san/00/15201/san/0121.htm

10- Maita Veliz L, Ramos Perfecto D, Maita Castañeda L M, Gálvez Calla LH. Necrotizing periodontal diseases Part I. Odontol. Sanmarquina [journal on the Internet] 2014. [cited 10 March 2018]; 17(1):35-39. Available from:

revistainvestigacion.unmsm.edu.pe/index.php/odont/article/view/9768

11- Benito Urdaneta M. Oral manifestations in HIV-positive patients and their relationship with CD4 lymphocyte values. Act Odont Ven [Journal on the Internet] 2007. [cited 17 March 2018]; 45(2):1-7 Available from:www.actaodontologica.com/ediciones/2017/2/manifestaciones_bucales_pacien tes_vih_positivos.asp

12- Expósito Delgado AJ, Vallejo Bolaños E, Martos Cobo EG. Oral of HIV infection in childhood: review article. Med Oral Patol [Journal on the Internet] 2004. [cited 17 March 2018]; 9:410-20. Disponible en:scielo.isciii.es/scielo.php?script=sci_arttext&pid=S1698- 44472004000500006

13- Rodino Perri, A. Audiovisual media and their use in distance learning. [monograph on the Internet] .Costa Rica: Universidad estatal a distancia. 2017. [cited 17 March 2018]. Available from: https://books.google.com.cu/books?id=xC7iIzBl8pkC&pg=PA120&lpg=PA120&dq=Los+medios+audiovisuales+y+y+su+uso+en+la+ense%C3%B1anza+a+distancia.+Costa+Rica:+University+state+to+distance&source=bl&ots=Zt4OkFn2dY&sig=bxFxoHvw3QuI32y6yRSYgMoo9Wk&hl=en- 419&sa=X&ved=2ahUKEwiFj-W_5lHeAhWQpFkKHQ-JDPEQ6AEwAnoECAcQAQ#v=onepage&q=Los%20medios%20audiovisuales%20y%20su%20uso%20en%20la%20ense%C3%B1anza%20a%20distancia.%20Costa%20Rica%3A%20Universidad%20estatal%20a%20distancia&f=false

14- Estevez Solano.R, Bravo de las Casas.M. Design of an educational software for the prevention of sexually transmitted infections. SIDASTUDI.2009.

[cited 6 Mar 2018]. Disponible en:http://www.sidastudi.org/es/registro/d25f08042482367a01269a9547db0363

15- Monteagudo Medrano K. Educational software to contribute to the prevention of STI/HIV/AIDS in adolescents in Cifuentes.2017 [cited Mar 6, 2018]. Available fromwww.enfermeria2017.sld.cu/index.php/enfermeria/2017/paper/download/188/36

BIBLIOGRAPHY .

EMPLOYED FOR THE CONFECTION OF THE EDUCATIONAL HIPERENTORNUM Estom-VIHSoft.

1- Collective of authors. Manual de Bioseguridad Estomatológica. Havana: Editorial Ciencias Médicas, 2007.

2- Collective of authors. Compendium of Periodontics. 2nd ed. Havana: Editorial Ciencias Médicas,2017.

3- González Naya G, Montero del Castillo ME. Comprehensive General Stomatology Havana: Editorial Ciencias Médicas,2013.

4- Santana Garay, J. C. HIV infection in the oral complex. Havana: Editorial Ciencias Médicas, 2000.

5- Collective of authors. Programa Nacional de Atención Estomatológica a la Población. Havana: Editorial Ciencias Médicas,2017.

6- Alemán Miranda O, Jardón Caballero J, Domínguez Y. Oral conditions related to HIV/AIDS. [monograph on the Internet]. Madrid: Editorial Academica Española ;2017. [cited 17 March 2018]. Available from: https://www.amazon.es/Afecciones-bucodentales-relacionadas-VIH-SIDA/.../3330091.

7- Alemán Miranda O, Domínguez Y, Aput A. Biosafety in HIV/AIDS. [monograph on the Internet]. Madrid: Editorial Academica Española ;2017. [cited 10 March 2018]. Available at: https://www.amazon.es/Bioseguridad-SIDA- Otto-German-Miranda/dp/6202249889.

8- HIV and AIDS. Statistical data. Infomed. 2017. [cited 17 March 2018]. Available from: http://temas.sld.cu/vihsida/informacion-basica/sobre-vih-y- aids/statistical-data/summary-2017/.

9- Santana Garay JC. Atlas of pathology of the oral complex. 2ª.ed. Havana: Editorial Ciencias Médicas, 2010.

10- Alemán Miranda O, Jardón Caballero J, Domínguez Y. Infectology and parasites in Stomatology. [monograph on the Internet]. Madrid: Editorial Académica Española ;2017. [cited 10 March 2018]. Available from: https://www.amazon.es/Infectología-y-parásitos-en

Estomatología/dp/6202235594

11- Donado Rodríguez M, Martínez-González JM. Oral Surgery. Pathology and Technique 4th ed. Spain: Elsevier, 2014.

12- Maita Veliz L, Ramos Perfecto D, Maita Castañeda L M, Gálvez Calla LH. Necrotizing periodontal diseases Part I. Odontol. Sanmarquina [journal on the Internet] 2014. [cited 10 March 2018]; 17(1):35-39. Available from:

revistainvestigacion.unmsm.edu.pe/index.php/odont/article/view/9768

13- Murillo Ladinez N Y. Acute Ulcerative Necrotizing Lesions and their relationship HIV/AIDS [doctoral thesis]. Guayaquil: University of Guayaquil. Pilot Faculty of Dentistry ;2014.

14- Benito Urdaneta M. Oral manifestations in HIV-positive patients and their relationship with CD4 lymphocyte values. Act Odont Ven [journal on the Internet]. 2007 [cited 17 March 2016]; 45(2):2. Available from:www.actaodontologica.com/ediciones/2017/2/manifestaciones_bucales_pacientes_vih_positivos.asp.

15- Expósito Delgado AJ, Vallejo Bolaños E, Martos Cobo EG. Oral manifestations of HIV infection in childhood: review article. Med Oral Patol [journal on the Internet]

2004. [cited 17 March 2018]; 9:410-20. Available from: scielo.isciii.es/scielo.php?script=sci_arttext&pid=S1698- 44472004000500006

16- Gallardo-Rosales R, Castillo-Torres K, Alegría-Conejeros P, Blackburn- Tapia E. Oral manifestations in HIV/AIDS patients at Hospital Base de Valdivia in Chile. Rev CES Odont [journal on the Internet] 2016.[cited 17 March 2018]; 29(2): 12-19. Available lnwww.scielo.org.co/pdf/ceso/v29n2/v29n2a03.pdf

Annex 1 Knowledge survey. Mark with an X the correct answer

1- Angular stomatitis manifests clinically as fissures or cracks that affect:

a--- corner of the mouth. b--- palate.

c--- floor of the mouth. d--- tongue.

e--- buccal mucosa.

2- The main oral manifestations of AIDS are: a-____candidiasis
b- _ hairy leukoplakia
c- __ chronic fibrous gingivitis
d- _ necrotizing gingivitis
e- _Kaposi's sarcoma
f- _non-Hodgkin's lymphomas.
g- _Hard chancre

3- A 30-year-old male patient with a diagnosis of HIV-positive who went to the dentist for a periodic check-up. During the intraoral examination, 36 was detected with loss of vitality and coronary destruction, so it was decided to extract the tooth. While performing the procedure the stomatologist cuts himself during the sindesmotomy. Mark with an X the immediate treatment to the exposed area.

---- Wash the wound or puncture with soap and water (do not apply disinfectants such as hypochlorite or squeeze the lesion).

---- Wash affected mucous membranes with plenty of water.

---- Wash the wound or puncture with soap and water. Then apply disinfectant substances on the wound.

__ Clean the wound with gauze soaked in sodium hypochlorite and then cover the wound.

4- Check V or F as appropriate.

___ Kaposi's sarcoma is a malignant tumor of the lymphatic endothelium caused by the human papillomavirus. It presents intraorally.

___ Diffuse undifferentiated non-Hodgkin's lymphoma is a malignant disease associated with HIV. Most are of B-cell origin and Epstein Barr virus is found in the cells several cases.

_____ Hairy leukoplakia is treated at the first level of care.
___ The most common pediatric alterations in the oral complex due to HIV infection lichen planus and oral candidiasis.

Mark with an X the correct answer

5- Among the universal precautions that the stomatologist must comply with to avoid contagion are:

___ Avoid skin or mucosal contact with blood and other universal precautionary fluids in all patients by means of protective barriers.

_____ Hand washing.

_____Use of gloves (never a substitute for hand washing).

_____Use of caps in surgical areas.

_____ Use of boots in surgical areas.

_____ Avoidance of occupational accidents.

_____ Attach the cap to the needle after finishing.

6- HIV is a disease that is currently plaguing mankind, with its incidence increasing over the years. To prevent the proliferation of this disease we can:

_____Abstinence

_____Monogamy

____ Know the habits, customs and sexual behavior of the partner before initiating sexual relations.

_____Having an active and unprotected sex life

___ Once a stable relationship is achieved, abandon the use of condoms.

7- The routes of HIV transmission are:

_____Sexual

_____Blood

_____ Perinatal

_____ Contact with saliva

_____Digestive

_____ Respiratory

8- Relate the items in column A to those in column B.

A B

1- AIDS

_____Koplik stains
_____ Wickham's striae.
_____Necrotizing Periodontitis
_____Hutchinson Triad
_____ Linear gingival erythema

Annex 2. Questionnaire.

Please answer the following survey with the utmost sincerity. The survey is anonymous and confidential, so we count on your cooperation for the development of our research.

The objective of the same is the creation of a didactic material to support teaching and we would like to know which of the following options you would prefer to receive information related to HIV-AIDS and its relation to stomatological practice

_____educational hyperenvironment

_____Audiovisual program

_____Websites

_____Powerpoint with hyperlinks

Annex 3. Questionnaire for product evaluation by specialists.

I am writing to you to request your collaboration for your professional competence and to put for your consideration the following material considered an educational hyperenvironment. We appreciate your attention and the help provided, which will be very useful in our current work.

Name and ____

Institutio____

Graduated ____

Position ____

Category ____

Category ____

Mark with an X the evaluation you give to the variables mentioned below after having interacted with the educational hyperenvironment:

1- Presentation Quality

----High ------Medium -------------Low

2- Quality of production

----High ------Medium -------------Low

3- Scientific quality

----High ------Medium ------------ Low

4- Practical Utility

---- Total ----- Partial -------------- None

Other criteria that you consider may contribute to improve the quality of the product:

Annex 4.

Questionnaire on students' opinion about the quality and usefulness of the product.

1- How did you find the Estom-VIHSoft educational hyperenvironment helpful in integrating knowledge?

Tota_

Partia_

Does not ____________

2- The quality of the images, videos and sound simulations was: _

Medi_

Downloa__________

3- Do you consider Estom-VIHSoft to be easy to use? Tota_____

Partia_

Does not provide _____________

4- The design and colors were? Adequat___

Moderately _________________________

Inadequat_______________

5- Do you accept this didactic product as a teaching aid in support of teaching activities?

Accepted________________ Not __________

6- Were you motivated by the product?

Yes_ No _______

7- Your understanding of the product content was: _

Moderately ___________________

Inadequat__________

ANNEX 5

Endorsement of Estom-VIH-Soft application

We hereby state that the hyperenvironment has been successfully applied in the Faculty of Stomatology of the University of Medical Sciences of Santiago de Cuba, proving its affordability and usefulness through a study conducted with 5th year students of Stomatology.

____

Dr. Lizel Diaz del Mazo

Dean Faculty of Stomatology of Santiago de Cuba

Annex 6. Informed Consent

I hereby affirm that after being informed by the Head of the Department of General Comprehensive Stomatology of the School of Stomatology of the objectives of this research I agree to participate in it knowing that:

The study will not affect my psychological and physical integrity; my participation will serve to improve the quality of teaching in the career of Stomatology.

Name and ____

Dat__

ANNEX:7

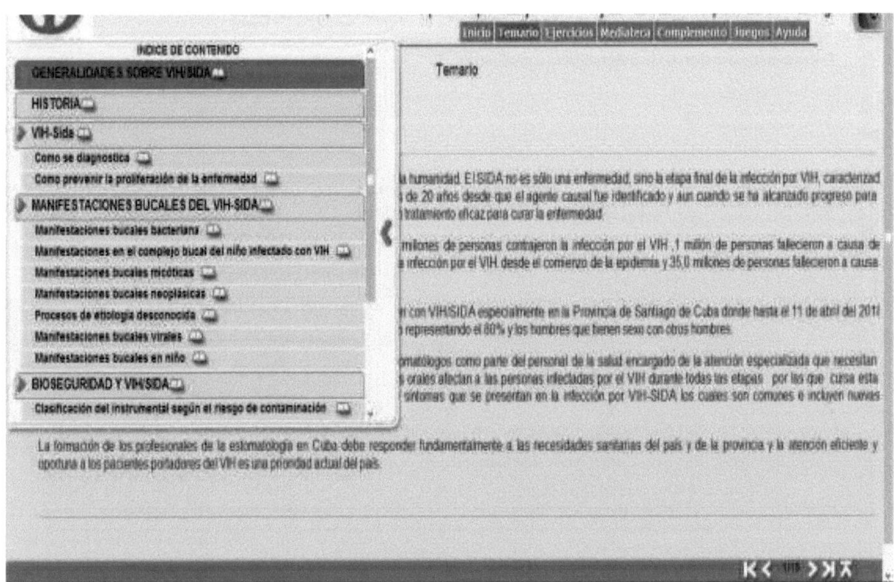
Inicio | Temario | Ejercicios | Mediateca | Complemento | Juegos | Ayuda
INDICE DE CONTENIDO
GENERALIDADES SOBRE VIH/SIDA
HISTORIA
VIH-Sida
Como se diagnostica
Como prevenir la proliferación de la enfermedad
MANIFESTACIONES BUCALES DEL VIH-SIDA
Manifestaciones bucales bacterianas
Manifestaciones en el complejo bucal del niño infectado con VIH
Manifestaciones bucales micóticas
Manifestaciones bucales neoplásicas
Procesos de etiología desconocida
Manifestaciones bucales virales
Manifestaciones bucales en niño
BIOSEGURIDAD Y VIH/SIDA
Clasificación del instrumental según el riesgo de contaminación
Temario
La formación de los profesionales de la estomatología en Cuba debe responder fundamentalmente a las necesidades sanitarias del país y de la provincia y la atención eficiente y oportuna a los pacientes portadores del VIH es una prioridad actual del país.

ANNEX:8

El reconocimiento temprano, el diagnóstico y el tratamiento de las lesiones orales asociadas a la infección por VIH pueden reducir la ______

La candidiasis ______ y ______

Las manifestaciones orales relacionadas con el SIDA pueden clasificarse en ______

En el manejo de las personas expuestas a sangre o fluidos potencialmente contaminados el primer paso a seguir es ______

El periodo de incubación del VIH puede extenderse hasta ______

Las gafas protectoras deben ser ______ y ______ al rostro y han de ______

En el grupo de las neoplasias, la más relacionada con el VIH es ______

El deterioro de los guantes, se produce por el empleo de agentes ______ , ciertas lociones de base de aceite o el calor, como la autoclave.

Se recomienda mantener las agujas dentro de su tapa durante el tratamiento y también la realización de la ______ durante el uso del instrumental de tartrectomía.

Los dientes extraídos para ser usados en la docencia a los alumnos de estomatología, deben considerarse ______ porque contienen sangre y toda persona que los transporte debe tener el cuidado necesario.

Previo a cualquier manipulación docente por los estudiantes, los dientes extraídos deben ______ con detergente y agua, o con un ______ posteriormente se sumergerán en una solución fresca de hipoclorito de sodio al 1:10 u otro líquido germicida; las personas que realicen estas manipulaciones siempre deben usar guantes y tomar todas las medidas conocidas y presentadas para evitar la contaminación.

En Cuba existe un Programa de intervención educativa dirigido a personas que viven con VIH que tiene como título ______ el cual cuenta de ______ encuentros distribuidos por temáticas.

Como objetivo ______ del Programa de intervención educativa dirigido a personas que viven con VIHD se encuentra demostrar la importancia de conocer los aspectos esenciales de esta entidad patológica que afecta ______

Las pruebas que se realizan para hacer un diagnóstico de VIH detectan los anticuerpos que el organismo produce como respuesta ante tal infección. En CUBA se realizan dos tipos de pruebas ______ y ______

ANNEX:9

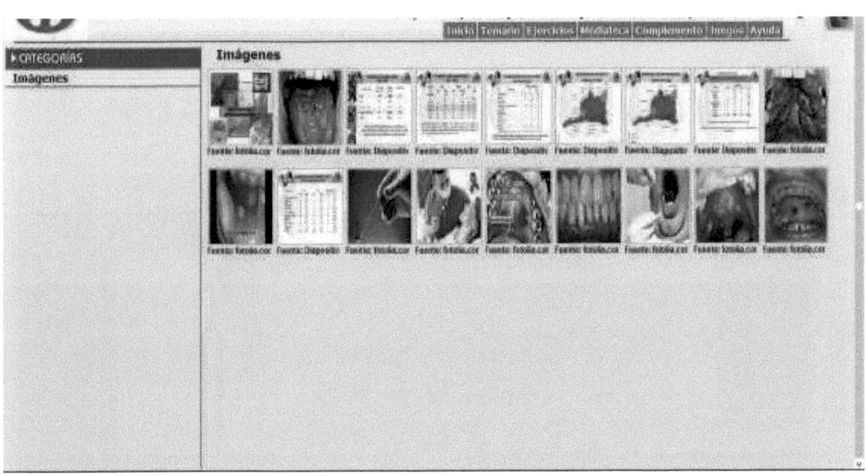

Inicio Temario Ejercicios Mediateca Complemento Juegos Ayuda
CATEGORÍAS
Imágenes
Imágenes

ANNEX:10

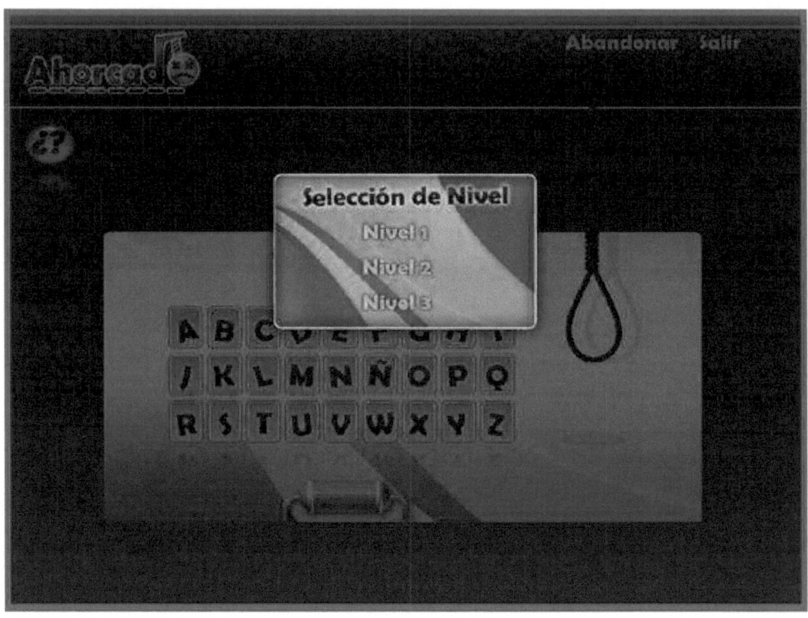
Ahorcado
Abandonar
Salir
Selección de Nivel
Nivel 1
Nivel 2
Nivel 3
A B C
J K L M N Ñ O P Q
R S T U V W X Y Z

FSC
www.fsc.org
MIX
Papier aus verantwortungsvollen Quellen
Paper from responsible sources
FSC® C105338

Printed by Books on Demand GmbH, Norderstedt / Germany